I0072393

Empower

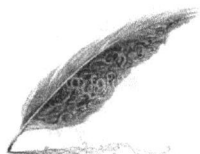

Publishing

Eldon S. Beard, MD

Also from
Eldon S. Beard

Refiner's Fire:
The Building of Faith Through Affliction

and *Empower Publishing*

MEDICINE IN AMERICA

ELDON S. BEARD, MD

Edited by Dr. Linda Felker

Empower Publishing
Winston-Salem

Eldon S. Beard, MD

Empower

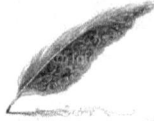

Publishing

Empower Publishing
302 Ricks Drive
Winston-Salem, NC 27103

First Empower Publishing Books edition published
July, 2024
Empower Publishing, Feather Pen, and all production design are trademarks.

For information regarding bulk purchases of this book, digital purchase and special discounts, please contact the publisher at publish.empower.now@gmail.com

Cover design by Eldon S. Beard

Manufactured in the United States of America
ISBN 978-63066-606-4

Table of Contents

Eldon S. Beard, MD

Dedication

First, I want to thank Dr. Linda Felker for her invaluable help in bringing this book to publication.

I want to thank my medical school instructors for providing a quality medical education and allowing room for God to be involved in the medical process.

To my beloved wife, Pam, who has supported me through our lives together and during the writing of this book.

To my friends and pastors at The Crossing Church for support and spiritual guidance over the past 6 years.

Most of all, to my Lord and Savior Jesus Christ, who not only saved my soul, but gives me guidance day by day in my personal and professional life. To Him be the Glory and Honor forever!

Eldon S. Beard, MD

Foreword

In my book, "Refiner's Fire. The Building of Faith Through Affliction," I explained that medicine in America has undergone a transformation, and not for the better. When I first began practicing medicine, virtually all physicians' offices were owned by the physicians practicing in them.

Over the course of my career, most physicians have become employees of hospitals or corporations which own the practices. I saw many of the traditional medical offices being purchased by hospitals. I have been congratulated by pharmaceutical representatives who visit our office for maintaining a solo family practice.

I practice medicine in a very competitive environment in terms of competition from the corporate entities. We probably have the highest ratio of physicians to patients of any place I know.

Because of the competition from these corporate entities, maintaining my practice has felt much like trying to keep an overloaded airplane flying with one engine out. Indeed, I have taken almost no income from the practice for a year or so, only being able to maintain salaries for my staff and pay the office expenses.

If I did not have my Social Security retirement

income, I would be destitute.

For the past 18 months I have been exploring alternative employment, but nothing has materialized, I thought my only option was to join the corporate world. Then last week I received a letter from a commercial realtor who was assisting a local physician in selling his practice. Initially, I tossed the letter in the trash, but as I contemplated it further, I thought, "God, maybe this is the way that You have planned to save my practice." It was as if God was saying, "OK, Eldon. You've tried things on your own long enough. Now try it **MY** way!"

I retrieved the letter from the trash and contacted the realtor. I met him with the physician at the doctor's office. It turns out I had shared call with him many years ago. We discussed the situation, and while it is unexplored territory for me, I firmly believe that this is my best path forward. As I begin this new undertaking, it will allow me to maintain my current practice while taking on a new patient population, generating greater income while maintaining the intimate relationship with my patients. It is a major undertaking, but I feel the same peace I felt when I first opened my private practice in 1987. My wife and oldest son are not exactly thrilled and I am somewhat apprehensive, but I am convinced that it is of God. I would appreciate your prayers as I begin this new undertaking. Just today I had a patient thank me for how I had helped her. I asked her, "What did I help you with?" She replied that I had helped her with the tremendous anxiety she had experienced over the years that no other physician had been able to help her with. There is nothing more rewarding for me than to have a patient thank me for helping them with their problem. This is the intimate relationship that I have with my patients.

As I embark on this new undertaking, I have contemplated what to write in this book, and my plan is to try to inform you about aspects of the health care system in America which will help you as you try to navigate this system.

Eldon S. Beard, MD

The Practice of Medicine

In America

I feel blessed to have had a quality medical education. One of my instructors taught us "we merely set the stage. God does the healing." In his book "Flying Closer to the Flame," Charles Swindoll describes healing for the Christian. He cites James 5:14-15.

Is anyone among you sick? Let him call for the elders of the church, and let them pray over him, anointing him with oil in the name of the Lord. And the prayer of faith will save the one who is sick, and the Lord will raise him up. And if he has committed sins, he will be forgiven.

He explained that in that day, the only medicine the priests had was oil. The medication did not really matter. The healing came from the Lord. I was with the Deacons in my former church as we prayed over a fellow Deacon who had an impossible medical problem which the doctors were unable to heal.

The pastor anointed him with oil. I admit to being amongst the "ye of little faith," and did not believe that our action would heal him. Within days we heard from our fellow Deacon that his condition was healed. That taught me to pray, "believing that what I desire has already been granted."

I believe that many of my patients have been healed, not because of any special abilities that I have, but because of my relationship with the Lord. Sometimes (not always), especially when I feel a patient's situation is particularly difficult, I offer up a quick prayer that God will guide me when dealing with their situation. He has never failed me in these situations.

Because I am the only physician in my office, I enjoy a very intimate relationship with my patients. We will often sit and chat about aspects of their lives other than their medical condition. They will ask how I am doing, and many say they pray for me. It deeply touches me when they tell me that.

I just saw a patient who said she thought about me yesterday. The thing that made her think of me was her Bible. Years ago, she was about to have heart surgery and she was very frightened. I shared Joshua 1:9 with her.

"Have I not commanded you? Be strong and courageous. Do not be afraid; do not be discouraged, for the Lord your God will be with you wherever you go."

This calmed her prior to her surgery. The day before she came to see me, she took her bible out. Her bible was open to Psalms, but the marker ribbon was in Joshua chapter 1. She smiled as she shared this with me.

My own experience with physicians when I have

been a patient has been rather pathetic. I remember taking a vacation to St. Simon's Island, GA in 1986. I experienced a heart rhythm called atrial fibrillation. I knew I was in it because of my rapid, irregular pulse.

Friends who were vacationing with us took me to a local physician who unfortunately misdiagnosed me despite having an EKG. He believed that I was in a rhythm called supraventricular tachycardia. I knew that this was incorrect because my rhythm was rapid and irregular. The rhythm in supraventricular tachycardia is rapid and **regular**.

He wanted to do a procedure called a "dive reflex" on me. The dive reflex occurs when a person submerges their face in water and holds their breath. It causes the heart rate to decrease and sometimes it can break supraventricular tachycardia (but **not** atrial fibrillation).

He proceeded to fill his sink with water and wanted me to put my face in it. I was reluctant, but didn't want to seem uncooperative, so I complied. It did not work as I had expected. I was relieved that he transferred me to the local hospital where I received proper treatment.

Over the past year I have had some medical problems including blood clots in my leg and lungs. We were at the beach, and it would have taken hours to go to a medical facility, so I called in blood thinners to a local pharmacy. My leg was better in 48 hours.

I often treat my own medical situations when I can. My wife asked me why I did not see a doctor about the blood clots, and I told her that there was nothing left to do except wait for the blood thinners to do their job.

I went to an urgent care when we returned home to try to get some medication for the pain. They refused and said that I needed to have tests to check for the condition. Thanks for the help!

When my wife tells me to go see a doctor for something that requires minor treatment like a cough or cold, I tell her (I am not being conceited when I say this), "No, because I'm the best doctor I know!"

This is borne out by the fact that I was in atrial fibrillation again after my blood clots. I knew that I could not treat this on my own. I made an appointment with a cardiologist near my home. I explained that I hoped to get clearance for some elective surgery before the end of the year. (This was in November) He ran some blood work, did an echocardiogram, changed some of my medication, and told me to come back in three months!

I received a call from his nurse who told me that if my pulse went below 50 beats per minute, he wanted me to increase the dose of a medication which is designed to slow your heart rate. I asked if she was sure, and she replied in the affirmative. I asked if she would please double check and she agreed.

The message was supposed to be if my heart rate was **above** 50 beats per minute I should increase the medication. I was able to pick up on this mistake, but someone with no medical training would be at the mercy of these people!

Upon getting my test results, the cardiologist

sent word to me through his office staff that I should go immediately to the emergency room. I asked why and was told that I was in heart failure and renal failure and needed immediate treatment.

I told them that I did not feel bad and questioned why I needed to go to the emergency room. They were insistent over the next few days, so I capitulated and went to the emergency room on a Friday afternoon. I spent the first 30-45 minutes trying to explain why I was coming to the emergency room. The only answer that I could give them was that my cardiologist insisted that I come to the ER.

The diagnosis of heart failure was made based on a measure on the echocardiogram called, "ejection fraction." The problem with this is that this measure is inaccurate when a person is in atrial fibrillation.

Likewise, the diagnosis of renal failure was based on my renal functions being elevated which also happens in atrial fibrillation because the heart is not efficient at pumping the blood around in that rhythm. I felt sure that if he would simply treat my atrial fibrillation all these parameters would improve.

They finally decided to place me on medication by IV to try and slow my heart rate. (It was running 150-160, with normal being 60-80.) They kept me on the medication by IV overnight without any appreciable reduction in my heart rate.

The next morning the on-call cardiologist (not my cardiologist), announced that the medication was having a detrimental effect on my heart's ability to contract. He stopped the medication.

Eldon S. Beard, MD

The cardiologist recommended that we should try a cardioversion, which is a procedure where they shock your heart to get it back into a normal rhythm. This is like rebooting or restarting a computer when it malfunctions.

He explained that the procedure would be more effective if I was on a particular medication for a couple of weeks before the cardioversion. He then said he wanted me to stay in the hospital for the rest of the weekend and have the procedure on Monday! (Where do they **get** these people!)

I explained that I was not going to sit in the hospital all weekend just to have him do a procedure that was unlikely to hold. I said, "I have tickets to the Trans-Siberian Orchestra tomorrow, and I am **not** missing that!"

They finally agreed to send me home on the medication and gave me my first dose before I left the hospital. I felt dizzy when I arrived home, so I laid down on the bed. I got up from the bed to go to the bathroom, and suddenly just dropped to the floor.

I was on several medications for high blood pressure. I stopped all of them and my top blood pressure number did not get above 100 for three days (normally 120-140). I went back to my cardiologist, and he decided to go ahead with a cardioversion. It took him three tries and it held for less than 24 hours.

I felt that I was getting nowhere with this guy, so I called a cardiologist that I have known and shared patients with for many years. Initially, I was told that he had no open appointments until after the first of the year, but I was thrilled when his office called back and said he had an open appointment the next week.

He approved my surgery and told me that he wanted to admit me to the hospital after the first of the year to start a medication and do a cardioversion. The reason they admit you to the hospital to start you on the medication is that a small percentage of patients develop a fatal arrhythmia when started on it. (YIKES!)

I found it extremely interesting the way he put it. He wanted to schedule me to go into the hospital on a weekend when he was on-call because he did not want to "inflict" any of his colleagues on me.

He admitted me to the hospital and the cardioversion was successful. Then, he scheduled me for a follow-up visit with his Nurse Practitioner. When I saw her, she began to read notes which sounded like the cardiologist had written to her, but which included some things that he had never discussed with me.

One of them was that he didn't think that they should start me on a particular medication for heart failure because he thought that it might drop my blood pressure too low. Another was that he wanted to do something called an electrophysiologic study on me within a few months.

We had never discussed any of that. All the while she stared at her computer screen and banged away on the keyboard as though she was writing a novel on me. So, what does she do? She decides to put me on the medication the cardiologist had recommended against!

It was against my better judgment to do so, but I did not want to appear to be an uncooperative patient, so I complied. My top blood pressure number hovered around 100 for four days. On day five, I felt extremely dizzy, and my top blood pressure number was 77.

I sent a message to her through the patient portal, and I received a response from her to stop the medication (like they had to tell me!). I took the liberty of stopping the powerful fluid pills that I was taking. I was convinced that I was no longer in "heart failure" since I was back in a normal rhythm.

They had a bit of difficulty as they started me on the medication in the hospital because my blood sodium level was quite low, and that was a problem with the new medication. One treatment for low blood sodium is to restrict a patient's fluid intake to about a quart a day, so that was my instruction when I left the hospital.

I saw the Nurse Practitioner in follow-up, and she was surprised to hear that I had stopped all those medications. She exclaimed, "No one told **me**!" (read the chart, lady!) She said, "Well we need to get you on **something** for heart failure" and suggested another medication.

I told her, "You **do** realize that you have never done an echocardiogram on me when I **wasn't** in atrial fibrillation, don't you?" She acted perplexed for a moment and asked me if I had been drinking my full sixty-four ounces of fluid per day. I looked at her and asked her, "You **do** remember that I was sent home on fluid restriction, don't you?"

She again looked perplexed and I said, "Look, how about you do an echocardiogram on me before you try to put me on any more heart failure medications?" to which she replied, "Well, if you want to direct your own care!" I replied in frustration, "I don't want to direct my own care, but I **do** want to be treated appropriately."

I think people like this think, "He's **just** a family physician" as if I do not know anything about cardiology. Family physicians have broad training in all areas of medicine including pediatrics, internal medicine, and OB/GYN.

There is a running joke amongst the internal medicine specialists that family physicians learn less and less about more and more so that eventually they know absolutely nothing about everything, while specialists learn more and more about less and less so that eventually they know absolutely everything about nothing at all.

The Nurse Practitioner decided to yield to my wishes and I had my echocardiogram. I followed up with her the next day and she scheduled a follow-up visit with my actual cardiologist. (Thank **God**!) If I have this much trouble navigating the medical system, I worry about what the average patient must go through!

I had a discussion with my accountant about all the difficulties I had been having. She said that her mother used to fall down every time she stood up and she was on the same medication I was taking when I had my drop attack after my hospitalization. She said it took her and her mother years to convince her doctors that it might be her medication before they finally took her off of it.

When they finally stopped the medication, her mother stopped falling. My only advice to you is that you should not take everything your doctor says as the gospel. She had an instinctive and observational knowledge about her mother that the doctor who only saw her for **perhaps** 15 minutes (if she was lucky!) every three months did **not** have.

Part of the problem with the way we currently deliver healthcare in America is this corporate system which drives doctors to see as many patients as possible in as short a time as possible. Patients may see a different provider every time they go into the office. I have had patients who come to my office and complain about this very thing.

One of my long-term patients left my practice because his family thought he needed a younger doctor. He returned about a year later and said he went to see a doctor at his new practice. It was during the COVID-19 pandemic, so they did a COVID test. That test took ten minutes. When the doctor entered the room, he said, "Quick, tell me what is wrong with you! I only have five minutes!"

I had a patient come to my office recently that had had hernia surgery five days prior. He was having postoperative pain. He called the surgeon's office, and they told him to see his PCP!

This is a problem the **surgeon** should have dealt with! I tried to call the surgeon to speak to him about it. Years ago, when a physician was calling another physician, he was put right through to the other physician.

The entity I called used to have what they called the Physician Access Line (PAL) for just this reason. Instead of immediate access to the other physician, I got caught in an endless phone tree loop which provided no ability to identify myself as a physician.

I tried to call the PAL and ended up speaking to the front desk of the Family Practice department. She tried to connect me to the surgical department and ran into the same endless phone tree. The only options on the phone tree were "appointments" and "billing."

The corporate mode creates these huge entities where patients get swallowed up in the system. It is easy for employees to decide that they do not have to provide personal service to patients. My patient said he felt that the person's attitude toward him seemed to be, "I'm not going to do a **d**n** thing for you!"

How do we solve this problem? I have no definitive answers, but I do have some ideas. Somehow, we must convince large corporate entities that this is a horrible way to provide patient care. Make your voice heard. Complain when you feel mistreated or when you never seem to be able to see your PCP or when you can't be seen within 24 hours when you are ill.

When you **do** get to see your PCP, complain directly to them that you never are able to see him. If he cares, he will try to make some changes. If he does not, **move on**! Vote with your feet.

I have been appalled at times as my patients relate stories to me of treatment by other physicians. I wonder where these doctors got their training. I am reminded of the story of the woman who was healed by a touch of Jesus' garment when the passage says, "she had suffered at the hands of many physicians."

Finding a good physician is as difficult as finding a good church. These situations are similar in the fact that the good ones are unfortunately few and far between. If you have a good one, hang on to him. If you don't, ask your friends who they see and how much they like them.

I have wonderful and loyal patients. Many ask me if I plan to retire any time soon. I tell them that I cannot afford to retire, I owe too many people too much money. In reality, I **love** to practice medicine.

I believe the best doctors are the ones who truly love the practice of medicine. Ask your doctor how he likes the practice of medicine. If he tells you that he loves it, you have a good one. If he acts like, "Eh. It pays the bills," you may want to move on.

Health Insurance

There are basically two different types of health insurance in America. In the industry, insurance that is provided by your employer is called "commercial." Government provided programs are Medicare, Medicaid, and TriCare. TriCare is health insurance for people who are in the military or relatives of military personnel.

Medicare becomes mandatory at age 65, but some people can apply for it if they have certain medical conditions before age 65. I am no insurance broker, so if you want to know who can apply before age 65, speak to your insurance broker.

I have had patients say to me, "I can't wait until I get on Medicare so that I can get everything paid for!" I'm thinking to myself, "Buddy, you don't know what I know!" This is a good time for me to tell you about a nasty little secret that Medicare has if you do not already know about it. It is called the "doughnut hole."

This refers to the fact that Medicare will pay for your medications until you reach a certain spending threshold. Upon achieving this threshold, Medicare stops paying for your medications altogether and you are responsible for 100% of the cost. This is called "reaching the doughnut hole." Once you have paid a certain amount out of pocket, Medicare starts paying again. You have made it to the other side of the doughnut hole.

I had a patient come into my office in an extremely agitated state. His blood thinners (which are **imperative** for him to take!) had suddenly jumped astronomically in price. He stated that he was "offended" and refused the medication. I told him that he couldn't just stop them, so we made some other arrangements for him.

The pharmacist had tried to explain the doughnut hole to him, but he seemed unable to grasp the concept. I explained it to him again, and on finally comprehending the doughnut hole, he exclaimed, "Well **who** thought that up?!" You got it. Our wonderful Congress! I recommend that if you are purchasing a Medicare supplement, you get a plan that covers prescriptions. This should help you avoid the doughnut hole.

Medicaid is typically for low-income families and individuals who may have certain medical conditions which qualify them for it.

Insurance has evolved over time. I remember going to the doctor as a child. The doctor would write my mother a bill. I think the one I saw was $5. She then went out to the front desk and paid for it. The only insurance we had was what we called "hospitalization." As the name implies, it was only there in case you had to go into the hospital.

Medicine in America

If you are unhappy with your health insurance, we may only have ourselves to blame. Over time, patients wanted insurance to pay more and more of their medical bills. When I was a child, the arrangement between my doctor and my parents was simple. He provided a service, and my parents paid the bill. No middleman.

The system was simple and efficient. The doctor got his full fee and could decide what to charge each patient at his discretion without intervention by the government or the insurance company.

Now, the doctor must file a claim, wait to see how much the insurance company will pay (sometimes the insurance company may reduce the amount the doctor has filed by as much as half or more), then wait several days to several weeks to get paid. This tends to make the doctor charge more because of the reduction in his fee.

The people who really suffer because of this are the patients who do not have insurance. My office offers discounts to uninsured patients, but they still pay significantly more under this system, because fees are regulated by the government and the insurance industry. You cannot charge one patient one fee and another patient a different charge.

Over the course of time, patients wanted to have their prescriptions covered by insurance as well. The list of medications which your insurance will cover and at what level is called the formulary. Generally, formularies will have at least one medication in each category that it will cover.

Each medication is assigned to a tier. Most insurance plans have four tiers. Some have more. The higher the tier, the more expensive the medication. Tier 1 generally includes generic medications. Branded medications are assigned to higher tiers depending on what the insurance company has decided to pay.

Formularies generally change around the first of the year based on prices the insurance company has negotiated with the pharmaceutical companies. Patients may sometimes find they have to change their medication at the first of the year based on the new formulary. This is not a problem because the physician can prescribe an equivalent alternative medication.

Many insurance companies offer mail order prescriptions. Oftentimes these programs limit the quantity of medication a patient can get at their local pharmacy to a 30-day supply. They try to encourage patients to use the mail order service where the insurance company has more control over the price of the medication than they do at the local pharmacy.

Pharmaceutical companies often offer some of their most expensive medications through coupon programs. The patient can obtain medications, which may cost hundreds or even thousands of dollars per month, at a much-reduced cost or even for free. These programs are only available to patients with commercial insurance.

I asked a pharmaceutical representative why these programs are not available to patients with Medicare, Medicaid, and Tricare. I did not completely understand his explanation, but it had something to do with the government perspective that they were at a financial disadvantage with these programs. So, the pharmaceutical companies decided not to make these programs available to patients on government programs.

This also includes insurance obtained through the Healthcare Marketplace. Once again, the government has put you at a disadvantage! While the Affordable Healthcare Act (Obamacare) has made it possible for Americans to purchase health insurance at low cost, many of these plans have very high deductibles.

Before you purchase one of these plans, I would suggest that you calculate your yearly healthcare costs. If the premium plus deductible is more than your yearly healthcare costs, you may be better off to remain uninsured. Some physicians (me included) offer discounts to uninsured patients. Pharmaceutical companies offer patient assistance programs which provide free medication to patients who qualify financially. I have severe psoriasis which I have only been able to control with a monthly injectable medication. If I only had Medicare, the medication would cost $2500 per month. Because of the program from the pharmaceutical company and my coverage by my wife's insurance, the medication is free.

This emphasizes the contrast between government provided health coverage such as Medicare, Medicaid and Tricare and commercial insurance.

I will never forget years ago my physician wanted

me to have an MRI. My cost with insurance was $1400. I found out that if I had been uninsured, the radiologist would have discounted the cost of the procedure, and I would have paid only $1000!

Alternative insurance plans: Self- funded plans. These programs, such as Christian-based Medishare, take "premium" payments and place them in a fund. Members then make claims against the fund to pay for their medical costs. These plans also often let members participate in telemedicine, which allows them to do virtual medical visits.

I provide telemedicine visits, and once people try it, they often LOVE it! They are thrilled to find that rather than the typical 3-4 hour wait period at an Urgent Care facility (or even longer to be seen in the emergency room), they can have their problem resolved in a matter of minutes through a virtual visit. This is called "telemedicine."

If you desire to participate in telemedicine, I have a couple of recommendations.

- Obtain an electronic otoscope. These are available through Amazon for about $30. This device allows you to obtain a digital image of the inside of the ear on your smart phone. These images can then be uploaded for the physician to view. Without this, I cannot definitively diagnose an ear infection. I can merely recommend that you provide pain control.

- I would also recommend that you purchase rapid strep tests, also available through Amazon for about $30 for twenty-five tests. Without this, I can only rely on a set of screening questions to determine whether or not you may have strep. It may also prevent you from having to be seen, either virtually or in person, because if it is not strep, it is probably viral and will simply need to run its' course. I discovered the limitation of this series of questions (called Centor criteria) when a father called about his daughter who had a sore throat. According to the Centor criteria, his daughter had a low likelihood of having strep. It was then that the father informed me that he had already performed a strep test on his daughter and the test was positive. I said, "Sir, next time lead with that!"

- If you have typical flu-like symptoms (sudden onset of fever, body aches, fatigue, sore throat, malaise), make sure to call within 48 hours of onset of symptoms,

  because this is the critical time frame to initiate flu medication which may shorten the course of the illness by up to 24 hours.

- Buy an **accurate** thermometer. It is amazing how many patients call in and tell me they "felt feverish" because they did not have a thermometer. Fever (generally over 100.3) is an important determining factor in many disease states.

Concierge medicine. In this model, a physician takes direct payment from patients to provide ALL medical care. This may be paid annually or on a payment schedule. They typically do NOT file insurance claims.

The Explosion of Vaccination

In America

When I began my medical career, we vaccinated children against Polio, Tetanus (eventually evolving into Diphtheria, Pertussis [whooping cough] and Tetanus) (TdaP), Measles, Mumps and Rubella (MMR).

The polio vaccine is no longer recommended because the risk of complications from the vaccine outweigh the risk of getting polio, due to modern water treatment procedures.

We had illnesses which we felt to be normal childhood illnesses, which included chicken pox. Oftentimes, when a case of chicken pox was identified in the community, all the moms would bring their kids over to be near the sick child, so that their own child would be exposed to the sickness, and the child would also get chicken pox and get it over with.

When they developed the chicken pox vaccine, I never really recommended it to my patients because I feared that we would convert a relatively mild childhood illness into an illness which is much more severe in adults. This seems to have become the case.

In addition, the chicken pox vaccine is on my list of "lousy vaccines." It must remain frozen (-4 degrees Celsius) from the time it leaves the manufacturer until the time that it is administered to the patient. This presents significant logistical problems, with many opportunities for the vaccine to thaw out during shipment and once arriving at the provider's office.

When it first came out, it was said to be a "once in a lifetime" vaccine. (Heard that before) Now a booster is recommended at 4-6 years of age. Then they developed the first shingles vaccine which was basically an extremely high dose of the chicken pox vaccine.

I was at a medical conference where an infectious disease specialist from a major medical center was discussing the shingles vaccine. He said that the reason we had to vaccinate for shingles was that we were vaccinating for chicken pox. (A problem of our own creation?)

I told the speaker that I was not a big fan of the chicken pox vaccine and asked if he could he tell me why I should recommend the shingles vaccine to my patients. He replied, "Well, because it saves lives!" I'm sorry, but I have seen a lot of cases of shingles and have not seen anyone who looked to be near death! Perhaps it saves lives in individuals who are undergoing a bone marrow transplant or are in some other way compromised immunologically, but **not** in the general population.

I told him that my first wife, Vicki, had shingles when she was pregnant with Justin, and I had a case myself a number of years ago. It was more of a nuisance than anything else.

He went on to give an account about his children being vaccinated for chicken pox and developing chicken pox a year later, but he was sure that the vaccine had been mishandled at the pediatrician's office and had lost potency. (*HELLO! Dude you're making my case for me!*) He said that their chicken pox was less severe than it would have been if they had not been vaccinated. (*How do you know!?*) I wish I could have been inside the minds of the other physicians in the room as he unfolded his tale!

When I was a medical student, at-risk individuals were vaccinated for Hepatitis B. This included medical personnel and people exposed to blood and body fluids (IV drug users, people practicing "unsafe sex," etc.) Now the recommendation is for universal vaccination from childhood.

We used to vaccinate overseas travelers for Hepatitis A. Now the recommendation is for universal vaccination from childhood. There is also a pneumococcal vaccine recommended from childhood which used to be reserved for patients with respiratory or cardiac conditions and the elderly.

My current vaccination recommendations are Tetanus (Tdap) every 10 years. I personally take a flu shot every year. I never did this until I caught the flu as a resident doing a rotation in Clinton, NC. I was so miserable I wished someone would have just shot me to end my suffering! I had a horrible headache which nothing would alleviate. Laying my head on the pillow made it hurt worse. I ached all over. My hair (I had some at the time!) even hurt. I personally believe that the flu is worse than COVID.

I recently spoke to a woman on a telemedicine

call who described my exact same symptoms and she agreed with me.

There are two different pneumococcal vaccines, Pneumovax and Prevnar. The recommendation for Pneumovax is every five years for patients with cardiac or respiratory problems with only one dose given over the age of sixty-five. Prevnar is recommended in children starting at 6 weeks of age with no current recommendation for repeat doses.

Both vaccines are recommended in patients over sixty-five years of age, regardless of respiratory or cardiac status. If you are over sixty-five, you should get Prevnar first with Pneumovax administered one year later. The new shingles vaccine (Shingrix) requires two doses rather than one and has much more in the way of side effects than the previous vaccine.

I had a patient who participated in the trials for it and the first dose made her feel so bad she refused the second dose. The new shingles vaccine also carries a small risk of Guillain-Barre Syndrome. They throw this out cavalierly in the commercials.

Guillain-Barre Syndrome gained prominence during the swine flu vaccination programs of the 1970's because a significant number of patients receiving the vaccine developed it. Guillain-Barre Syndrome is also called ascending paralysis. This is because paralysis begins in the lower extremities and moves upwards. When the paralysis reaches the diaphragm, you must be put on a ventilator.

There is no known cure for Guillain-Barre Syndrome, but several treatments can ease symptoms and reduce the duration of the illness. Although most people recover completely from Guillain-Barre Syndrome, some severe cases can be fatal.

While recovery may take up to several years, most people are able to walk again six months after symptoms first start. Some people may have lasting effects from it, such as weakness, numbness, or fatigue. For these reasons, I do not recommend the shingles vaccine. I am reserving judgement on the RSV vaccine until we gain more experience with it.

I had three COVID vaccines and caught COVID twice. They tell you that the new vaccine is "updated," but it only covers the original strain and Omicron. It does not cover the current strain of COVID which is prevalent in the community. Personally, I am DONE with COVID vaccines! I will let you make your own decision about that!

There was a study in THE LANCET (A British medical journal) That showed that person actually was more likely to catch COVID in the immediate post-vaccination period. It was difficult to find, because the search engines were told by the powers that be to suppress it.

Common Misconceptions About

Disease States

Much of what I deal with in this chapter will have specific application to telemedicine. In telemedicine, patients have virtual encounters with a provider. They can get their problem taken care of in a 10–15-minute call as opposed to making an appointment to see a provider in person. When patients try it, they are usually thrilled.

Many patients that I speak to complain that their provider cannot see them for a week or more and there is a 3-4 hour wait at the local urgent care. The wait times at emergency rooms are even longer and you are exposed to all of the sickest patients as well.

As I outlined, several preparations can enhance your telemedicine experience: specifically, purchase of an electronic otoscope and home strep tests.

Apparently, there is no longer any such thing as the "common cold." Everyone has a "sinus infection." In reality, they usually have a viral upper respiratory infection or allergies. Usually, a sinus infection is characterized by nasal congestion lasting for ten days to two weeks and foul tasting or smelling drainage and/or pain in the upper teeth.

Medicine in America

When I was in training, I asked one of my instructors when they would prescribe an antibiotic for a patient with an upper respiratory infection (common cold). He replied, "If it has been five days and the patient is no better, I would start one."

In addition, we used to tell patients that greenish discoloration of their mucus indicated that they had a bacterial infection. Recent studies indicate that discoloration merely indicates inflammation, not infection.

Combine all of this with the advent of the Z-pack. A Z-pack is a 5-day course of an antibiotic called azithromycin. Many patients have been accustomed to receiving a Z-pack when they have a cold. The problem with this approach is that you only take the Z-pack for five days. The natural course of an upper respiratory infection is generally five to seven days. So, when the symptoms improve, patients assume that it was the Z-pack that cured the problem.

All of this combines to cause us to overprescribe antibiotics. Over time, this tends to create resistant organisms to the antibiotic. This necessitates the development of new antibiotics to which the organisms are not resistant.

One of the most common examples of this is MRSA. MRSA stands for Methicillin Resistant Staph Aureus. Staph aureus is a bacterium which naturally lives on your skin, and in normal circumstances actually protects your skin from more dangerous bacteria and fungal organisms.

Because of our overuse of antibiotics through

the years, we have selected out a strain of the organism which causes disease. It is for this reason that the telemedicine entity that I work for encourages us to avoid overprescribing of antibiotics. Many patients are QUITE unhappy when they do NOT receive their Z-pack.

Diabetes. "Doc, I don't understand! I do not eat any sugar!" Many diabetics don't realize that it is **carbohydrates** that matter. This includes starchy foods, like potatoes, dried beans, corn, pasta, bread, etc. A good rule of thumb is to mentally divide your plate in half. Half of the plate can be for non-starchy vegetables (broccoli, cauliflower, lettuce, greens, etc.).

Divide the remaining portion of the plate into quarters. One quarter is for protein (meat, fish, chicken, pork, etc.). The remaining quarter is for carbohydrates (potatoes, bread, fruit, etc.). Many diabetics think that they are eating healthy because they are eating a lot of fruit without realizing that the main nutritional value of fruit is carbohydrates.

Getting sick. Many patients believe that they became ill because they got chilled and then got overheated. One actually becomes ill because they have come into contact with germs. Colds are viral. They need to run their course. Antibiotics are ineffective against viruses.

I am reminded of the episode of "The Beverly Hillbillies" when Granny had a cure for the common cold. Mr. Drysdale was excited because he could see that this would be something from which he could make a lot of money. Mr. Drysdale caught a cold and Granny prepared the cure. Apparently, it tasted pretty foul based on the grimace on Mr. Drysdale's face as he took it. Granny declared, "Now in a week or ten days you'll feel right as rain!"

Special Considerations

In Geriatric Patients

I looked up the definition of geriatrics online and the definition which popped up said that it was the branch of medicine that dealt with old people. Whoever wrote that definition needs to be shot.

Specifically, geriatrics deals with patients over the age of sixty-five. Everyone ages differently. I have some patients in their nineties who could probably run circles around me and some around sixty-five who can barely move. The presence of medical conditions such as cardiovascular disease, lung disease, diabetes, high cholesterol, arthritis, and hypertension can affect a person's health and the pace at which they age.

While these can affect a person's health in the geriatric population, there are also changes specific to the aging process that can affect a person's health and well-being. Patients over sixty-five tend to have a less robust immune system and get sick more easily, become sicker with the illness, and recover more slowly than younger patients.

Many people do not realize how much our balance is dependent on pressure sensors in our feet. When a person is standing with their eyes open and then closes them, the pressure sensors are the main mechanism allowing a person to maintain their balance.

As we age, these sensors become much less sensitive. In a person whose pressure sensors are diminished or non-functional, they are very likely to be at risk of a fall when their eyesight is impaired.

Some situations which may arise include diminished eyesight (possibly due to cataracts) or a man getting up in the middle of the night because he must urinate more often due to an enlarged prostate. If he does not turn the light on, he highly likely could fall.

I used to fly down the stairs when I was in my twenty's and 30's. Now I must take each step slowly and carefully and use the handrail. There is a caricature seen often on TV and movies with the little old lady creeping along behind her walker. This really should not be something amusing to people. It is a serious situation. The fatality rate in elderly patients who fall and break a hip is **50%**!

There are several vaccines recommended for patients over sixty-five. It is recommended that all patients receive both pneumonia vaccines (Pneumovax and Prevnar) spaced a year apart, beginning with Prevnar. Shingles vaccine (Shingrix) is recommended, but I do NOT personally recommend it due to the reasons I have outlined previously.

Respiratory Syncytial Virus (RSV) vaccine (Beyfortus) is also recommended, but I am reserving judgment on this vaccine until we get more experience with it.

Dementia is common in the elderly. Some patients have mild symptoms which are controlled by medication and continue to work and function. I have a patient in his seventies who continues to travel around teaching seminars while another patient a couple of years younger than him must write all the instructions for how to take his medication down because he cannot remember from one moment to the next what I have just told him.

Dementia can be insidious. A person can function quite well when at home in their familiar environment and decompensate when they must be hospitalized. Several disease states can **mimic** dementia and must be ruled out when treating demented patients. Two of the most common are depression and hypothyroidism. Have your doctor check for these conditions before treating the patient for "dementia." When these conditions mimic dementia, it is called "pseudodementia."

Aging also causes loss of physical strength. I am fairly tall, so it is easier for me to rise and sit from a taller chair. I recently had a chair height toilet installed in my bathroom. If I go down on the floor, call a crane.

The skin tends to become drier as we age. To combat this problem, run a humidifier large enough to humidify your entire house during the winter months, to maintain a relative humidity of 30-40%. This will also help keep your mucous membranes moist.

As the mucus membranes of the upper respiratory tract dry out, they tend to crack, which will cause nosebleeds, and they become more susceptible to infection. Running a humidifier can actually help you to avoid catching colds and other upper respiratory infections.

Another way to combat dry skin is infrequent bathing. Most seniors only need to bathe two-three times weekly. If you have "problem areas," you can take care of these with what my mother used to call a "cat bath" and which my wife calls a "horse bath."

Constipation is a frequent problem in seniors. MiraLAX is a safe and effective laxative and can be used on a daily basis. Make sure that you maintain your schedule of colonoscopies based on your gastroenterologist's recommendations. Most gastroenterologists will discontinue colonoscopies on older seniors as the risk of the procedure exceeds the potential benefit in older patients.

I have touched on many aspects of aging in this chapter, but I have by no means covered the topic comprehensively. If you have questions about this or any other material I have discussed in this book, please feel free to contact me at eldonsbeard@gmail.com.

Telemedicine

This will be a short chapter. I want to talk a bit about this new telemedicine technology.

I started doing telemedicine a little bit a few years ago but got into it in earnest a year or so before the pandemic. This was **completely** God's timing. When the pandemic hit, office visits dropped to zero (my office manager stood guard and would not let anyone come into the office) and the telemedicine calls skyrocketed.

Before the pandemic, most patients would have to wait perhaps a few minutes to possibly up to an hour to speak to their care provider. During the pandemic, we could not keep up with the demand for telemedicine.

On the platform that I work with, we have a screen called the "Waiting Room." This is where patients are put in a queue to wait to speak to a physician. Encounters are coded white, green, yellow, and red. White means the patient has only been waiting a few minutes. Green means the patient has been waiting maybe 20 minutes or so. Yellow is next and then red. I am currently in the Waiting Room, and it is empty.

The online platform I use is not particularly busy this time of year. Calls sometimes become steady to always having at least a few patients in the Waiting Room during busy times of year, particularly the holidays. It can get fairly busy when families start taking vacation, as they can do a virtual visit rather than having to go to the local urgent care which is often booked up for 3-4 hours.

I rarely have a patient coded anything but white. During the pandemic, **all** calls were coded red, and it was not uncommon for patients to wait 24-36 hours for a call back. We could not keep up. The company offered additional cash incentives for each patient visit we did to encourage us to spend as much time online as possible.

I often performed consultations from home in the evenings. The income from telemedicine literally financially saved my practice. As I say, God's timing.

Telemedicine is great for patients who have simple problems, and most situations can be handled in a few minutes as opposed to waiting to get into urgent care. Most PCPs apparently do not leave slots in their appointment schedule to see sick, same day patients. (Although one of the local corporate practices is now advertising the fact that they have same day visits.)

Patients often call and say that they called their PCP and they could not see them for a week or more, even when they had an acute problem. People **love** telemedicine for this reason. It is an excellent platform. I feel that it is "the wave of the future."

Patients call and say that they complained about not being able to be seen, and someone told them about telemedicine. Some even say they knew that it was available through their health insurance (oftentimes at no additional charge) but never thought to use it until now.

Most patients are quite satisfied with how rapidly their problem can be handled. Some even get to make each call for free with no copay.

While it may be the newest, greatest thing since sliced bread, telemedicine has its limitations. We cannot examine the patient or obtain laboratory studies. This usually is not too much of a problem.

My instructors in medical school told me that I should already pretty much know what is going on with the patient before I examine them and run tests because of the medical history obtained from the patient.

I have found this to be quite true over the years. I will never forget what one of my instructors told me. He said," If you listen to the patient long enough, they will generally tell you what is wrong with them."

Because we cannot run tests in telemedicine, in order to treat strep throat, we must rely on a series of screening questions to try to determine the likelihood that a given patient has strep throat. This series of screening questions is called the Centor Criteria. It is based on symptoms, patient age, and other factors.

If you are going to participate in telemedicine, I have some suggestions that will improve your experience:

1. Purchase rapid strep tests. These are available through Amazon. Twenty-five tests run about $30.

2. Purchase an electronic otoscope. This device attaches to your smartphone and allows you to take digital images of the inside of your ear canal. Make sure to purchase one that allows you to save the images to your phone so that you can upload them to the telemedicine service. They also cost approximately $30.

3. Purchase an accurate blood pressure cuff, thermometer, and pulse oximeter. The pulse oximeter is the little clip-on thing the nurse puts on your finger when you go to the doctor these days. It will give you a blood oxygen level and take your pulse (as the name implies). These will allow you to take your "vital signs" to relay to the provider.

4. Most mild upper respiratory infections (common colds) last 5-7 days. You can wait a while on those. **However**, if you have typical flu-like symptoms (fever, scratchy or sore

throat, body aches, fatigue, nasal congestion, drainage) it is important to call immediately because there is a 48-hour window from the onset of symptoms in which medication can be started to shorten the duration of the illness for up to 24 hours.

Overall, telemedicine appears to be the newest evolution in healthcare delivery in American healthcare. Over time, I believe the American public will tend to embrace it.

The Pandemic

The first case of COVID-19 (officially designated SARS-CoV-2 [Severe Acute Respiratory Syndrome Coronavirus 2]) occurred in the city of Wuhan, China in December of 2019. The first Chinese death occurred on January 11, 2020. By mid-January 2020, infections were reported in Thailand, Japan, and Korea, all from people who had traveled to China.

On January 18, 2020, a 35-year-old man checked into an urgent care center near Seattle, Washington. He had just returned from Wuhan and had a fever, nausea, and vomiting. On January 21, he was identified as the first American infected with SARS-CoV-2.

In reality, dozens of Americans had contracted SARS-CoV-2 weeks earlier, but doctors did not think to test for a new type of virus. One of those unknowingly infected patients died on February 6, 2020, but her death was not confirmed as the first American casualty until April 21.

From the beginning, I have told people that COVID is the "new flu." It has been noted by some that many more people have been killed by the COVID pandemic than were killed in the original flu epidemic in 1918.

This is the difference between an "epidemic" and a "pandemic." COVID became a pandemic due to our increased mobility, sealing people in aluminum tubes in close proximity to one another and flying them all over the world. That is a perfect scenario for turning an epidemic (which COVID would have continued to be if travel to the area had been limited) into a pandemic.

In retrospect, everything the CDC told us about COVID turned out to be guesswork. I would not have a problem with that if they had just been honest with the American public and said, "Look. This is a brand-new disease. We are all learning as we go along.

Right now, these are our best recommendations. These recommendations are likely to change as we go along. We will keep you up to date as we gain new information."

Instead, they took the "expert" role and told us that this is what we needed to do and anyone who gave an opinion contrary to that was spreading "disinformation."

People were blocked on social media, reputations were ruined, some physicians lost their licenses. Anyone who had an opinion different from the "party line" was said to be against "science." Dictating an opinion to everyone is **not** science, it is the exact **opposite**. Science is the exploration of different possibilities to try and obtain the truth. Science is **not** governed by dictum.

At the time of the pandemic, the CDC's official definition of a "significant exposure" to COVID-19 was a total of 15 minutes in a 24-hour period within six feet of an actively coughing individual. During the shutdown, our church did not meet together, but I helped with the livestream.

I believe that I contracted COVID while doing that. It did not seem serious, mostly a bad cough. My wife had a cold and we tested her for COVID and she was negative, so I felt safe.

As I said previously, my office manager was controlling the door to our office like a guard dog, not letting anyone come to the office. We were obviously not seeing patients. My office space is perhaps sixty feet long by twenty feet wide. My office within that space is in the extreme rear of the building, while my office manager and nurse work in the extreme front of the building, separated by a double wall (there is an enclosed area between them housing the air handlers for the HVAC system). I stayed in my office, hacking away.

We worked from Monday through Thursday of the week, and on Thursday my office manager called the office and told my nurse that she felt **horrible**. We told her to come in to get a COVID TEST. She was positive for COVID.

Because of this, I told my nurse to check on herself. She too was positive, and of course, I was positive. So much for the CDC guideline. So much of what the CDC told us during the pandemic has been proven wrong that they have completely lost credibility with me.

Throughout my career, we have advised patients that natural disease imparted better immunity than immunization. Now with COVID that's different? I was astonished to learn that during the pandemic Pfizer actually had office space in the CDC building!

I don't have to tell you all of the ways society was damaged by the shutdowns. Businesses failed and churches failed. Children's education suffered. As a country, we have taken a blow. Many businesses and churches may never come back. Only time will tell how our children have been damaged.

But God is faithful. He can heal our greatest hurt, and He can heal us from this if we will only turn to Him.

Despite all the bad things that happened during the pandemic, some **good** things have actually come from it. I rarely go inside Sam's club anymore. I simply order stuff online, drive up, and they bring it out to my car. I have been an Amazon junkie for years. My motto is, "If Amazon doesn't have it, you probably don't need it!"

I have discovered Door Dash and Instacart. I do not mean to make light of the pandemic and all the hurt that it caused to so many people, but I believe we have "walked through the valley of the shadow of death" and have been seen safe on the other side.

FAQ's

Here are some subjects on which I am frequently asked questions:

1. **Hey, doc. When can I stop taking my blood pressure medicine?**

Many people don't understand that hypertension (high blood pressure) is a chronic illness. If you have it, you probably inherited it from your parents. Many people try to control their high blood pressure with diet and exercise.

Those are good things, but if you have hypertension, it is probably genetic and needs to be treated. Most people never realize that they have high blood pressure. For moderate elevations of blood pressure there are generally no symptoms. People do not experience symptoms like headaches unless they are in a hypertensive crisis.

A hypertensive crisis is a sudden, severe increase in blood pressure. The blood pressure reading is 180/120 millimeters of mercury (mm Hg) or greater. Long-term effects of hypertension which can be prevented with proper treatment include stroke, heart disease, kidney failure, and blindness. Some patients say, "But doc, I just don't like taking medicine." I ask them, "Would you rather take this pill, or have a stroke?" They generally opt for the pill.

2. Doc, is this place on my skin dangerous?

Fortunately, most of the skin lesions I check for people are benign lesions, seborrheic keratoses or pigmented nevi (common moles).

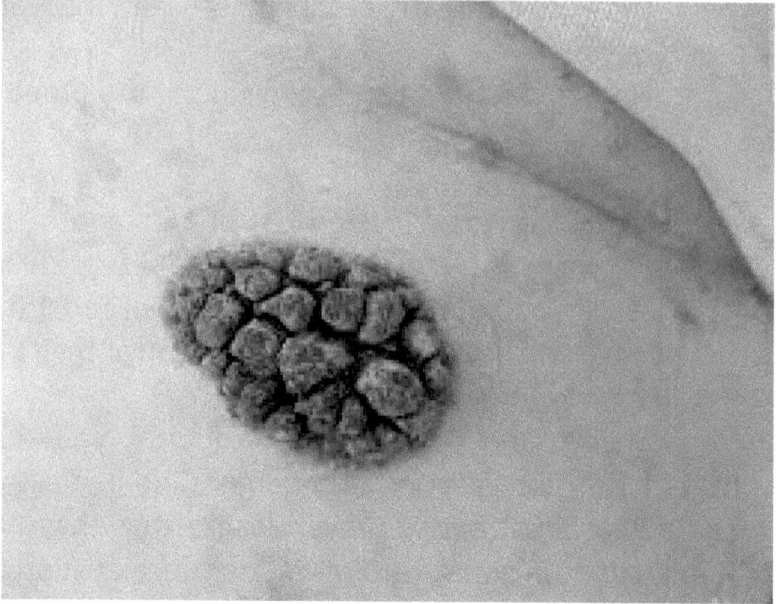

Seborrheic Keratosis

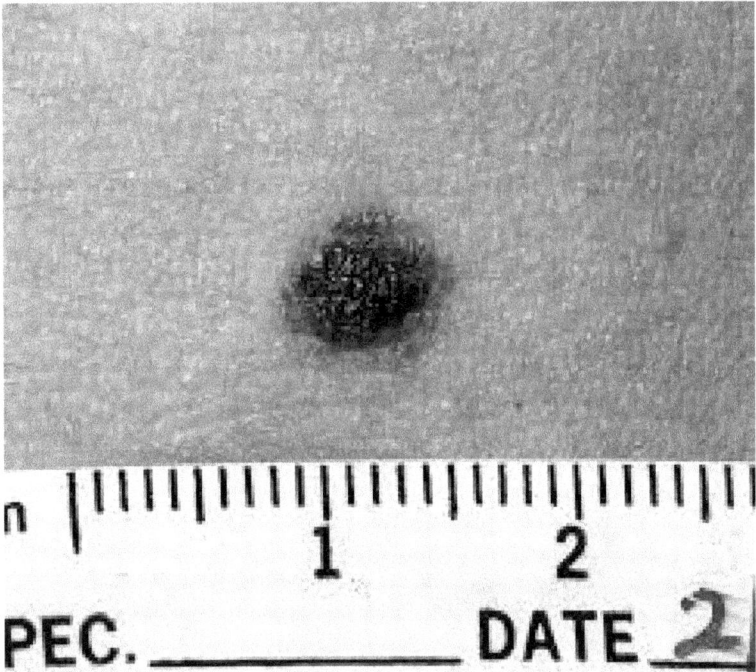

pigmented nevus

You can begin to evaluate your skin lesion by using the ABCs of dermatology.

- A: Area. Is the lesion larger than the size of a pencil eraser? It may be of concern.

- B: Border. Is the border smooth or irregular? An irregular border or a portion of the lesion growing outside of a regular border may be of concern.

- C: Color. Smooth brown coloration is usually not of concern. Irregular brownish coloration, or colorations of black or blue raise the concern of melanoma.

Other concerns would be a lesion that does not heal or that bleeds easily.

The main bad actors in skin lesions are squamous cell carcinoma, basal cell carcinoma, keratoacanthoma, and malignant melanoma.

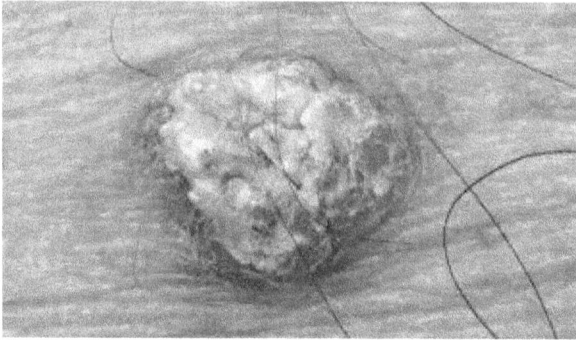

Squamous Cell Carcinoma

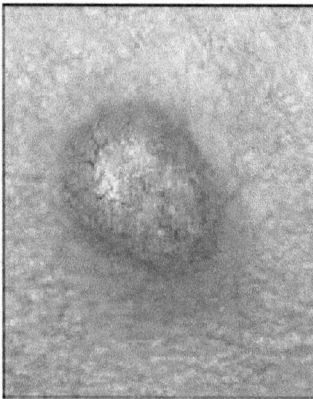

Basal cell carcinoma

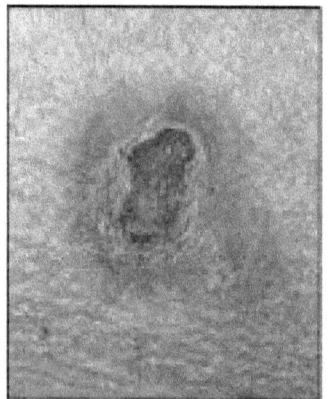

Squamous cell carcinoma

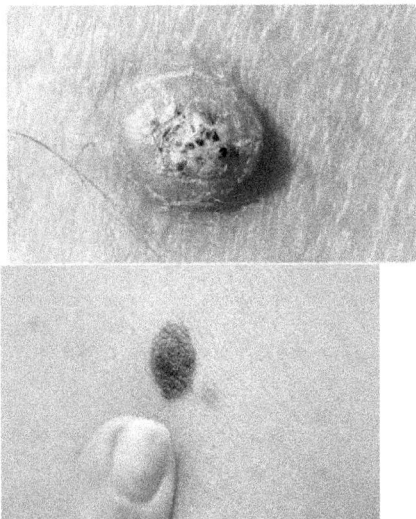

Keratoacanthoma and Melanoma

The **really** bad actor in the group is malignant melanoma. Removing a malignant melanoma in the earliest stage is crucial because unlike the other cancers, which are only locally invasive, malignant melanoma can metastasize (move to other areas of the body far removed from the original site of the lesion). If malignant melanoma metastasizes, it is almost universally fatal.

Early in my career, we did not consider keratoacanthoma a malignancy, but it was later been classified as a low-grade malignancy. All of the above skin lesions should be removed as soon as possible and sent for pathological evaluation.

3. Doc, what's this thing under my skin? Should

I have it taken out?

Lipomas are very common benign (not dangerous) tumors that grow just under the skin.

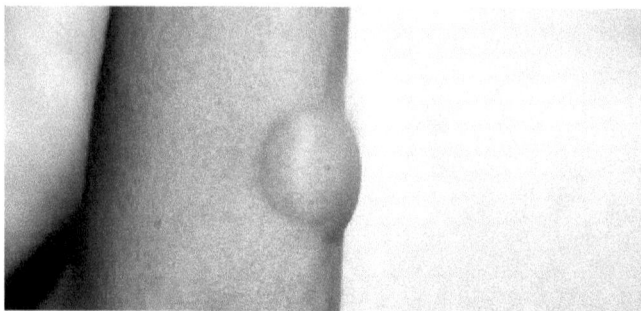

Lipoma

They tend to get larger over time. The only reason to remove them is if they are causing pain or if the patient just doesn't like the appearance. I had a very large one on the back of my head that made me look like I had another head, so I had it removed.

4. **Doc, when should I get a colonoscopy? Is there any alternative to a colonoscopy?**

Unfortunately, colon cancer seems to be on the rise, particularly among younger adults. I have a strong family history of colon cancer. When my father had colon cancer when I was in my forties. I began having colonoscopies and they found several polyps which, if left untreated, could become cancerous.

The previous recommendation was to have a screening colonoscopy at the age of fifty, but because of the recent rise of colon cancer in younger adults, the recommendation has been downgraded to age 45.

The one alternative to colonoscopy is a product called Cologuard. This is a stool DNA test which your doctor can order for you. A kit is shipped to your home, you follow the instructions in the kit for collecting the stool sample, and then you ship the kit back to the company.

It is considered an acceptable alternative to colonoscopy, but if it returns positive, you still must undergo colonoscopy.

5. Doc, this diabetes medication is so expensive. Can't I go back on my insulin?

I try my best to keep my Type 2 diabetics off insulin if it is at all possible. We have a great arsenal of medications to treat diabetes, but they tend to be pricey, and they are especially pricey for Medicare recipients. The reason I try to avoid insulin is the fact that while insulin lowers blood sugar, it also is lipogenic, meaning that it causes your body to produce fat cells.

When I explain this to patients, they are often willing to find a way to pay for the newer medications. Medicare is getting a little better about covering these new medications, but because of their high price, patients often reach their "doughnut hole" sooner.

6. Doc, why can't I get more than a 30-day supply of my medication at my local pharmacy?

This generally means that the patient has mail order pharmacy available through their insurance company. The insurance company wants patients to utilize the mail order pharmacy in preference to their local pharmacy because it gives them more control over drug prices.

Some patients are reluctant to utilize the mail order pharmacy, citing concerns about the security of their medication in the mail. I have used my mail order pharmacy for years and have had no problems whatsoever.

One caveat. Make sure that you have 7-10 days' worth of medication on hand when requesting refills to allow enough time for your mail order prescription to arrive.

7. Doc, what are the symptoms that a woman is having a heart attack? How different is it than a man's symptoms?

As with men, women's most common heart attack symptom is chest pain or discomfort. But women may experience other symptoms that are typically less associated with heart attack, such as shortness of breath, nausea/vomiting and back or jaw pain.

8. Doc, I am a professional person who has transitioned to being a caregiver at home. After five years, I find myself lonely, a little depressed, and tired. We planned and did all the right things to prepare for our senior years. But now all our plans are out the

window and I feel my life is upside down. What resources are there for caregivers like me?

One of the most important things for a caregiver is to be able to have a life outside the caregiving environment. Services such as Aging Care and Visiting Angels can provide these services for a fee. This allows you to remove yourself from the constant task of caregiving and "get a break from the routine."

I don't care how much you love your significant other, caring for them 24 hours a day seven days a week can get exhausting. You also can become isolated, which I believe is triggering your loneliness and depression. Seek the help of your physician about the possibility of taking medication for your depression.

I have had some in the Christian community resist antidepressant medication because they believe that if they just had enough faith, they wouldn't be depressed. That is far from the case. I believe that God has revealed the medications we have today to man for our good use. 2/3 of patients who go on antidepressant medication show improvement.

9. Hey, doc. Are these new weight loss drugs

safe and effective?

All the new once-weekly injectable medications were originally designed to treat Type 2 diabetes. They are all GLP-2 inhibitors (for Glucagon-Like Peptide inhibitors). Glucagon is a hormone in the body that increases blood sugar and speeds up your GI tract. Therefore, the GLP-2 inhibitors lower blood sugar and slow down the GI tract. A result of this is a decreased appetite. They **are safe and effective.** A major side effect is nausea.

If you don't have insurance coverage, these medications can cost around $500 per month. All weight loss drugs are designed to curb your appetite. If you can't afford them, all I can recommend is self-control. Don't load up your plate. Take small portions and eat slowly to allow your appetite to decrease.

Drink lots of water to give yourself a full sensation. A low carbohydrate diabetic diet is good for dieting. Eat small frequent meals throughout the day rather than one large meal.

In a study, they gave two groups the same number of calories to eat for the day. One group ate small frequent meals spaced throughout the day, while the other group ate one large meal. The group eating small frequent meals lost weight while the group eating one large meal gained weight.

Epilogue

In this book I have tried to give you some insight into the American medical system and some pointers which will help you to navigate it.

Our system is broken, that's for sure, but I believe in the transforming power of God and believe that He can help us even with this situation.

I would welcome any questions you might have. You can contact me at eldonsbeard@gmail.com.

In Christ,

Eldon S. Beard, MD

About The Author

Eldon Severin Beard, MD, is a Family Physician practicing in Winston-Salem, North Carolina. He and his wife Pam have a blended family with six children between them and eight grandchildren. They reside in Kernersville, North Carolina.

Pam works from home as a medical coder. She enjoys crafting and artwork. They have two dogs, Beau, and Bella. When people ask Eldon what kind of dogs they are, he says, "Heinz 57." (IYKYK)

In his spare time Eldon enjoys gardening and beekeeping. Both Eldon and Pam have a love for music and actually met in church choir. They attend The Crossing Church in Kernersville, NC, where Eldon is active with the Production Ministry running the computer for their live stream. He is also an active member of the Deacon Board and heads the church's Medical Ministry.

Check it out online at www.thecrossingnc.com.

www.ingramcontent.com/pod-product-compliance
Lightning Source LLC
Chambersburg PA
CBHW050514210326
41521CB00011B/2449